Peace Be With You

Peace Be With You

Peace Be With You

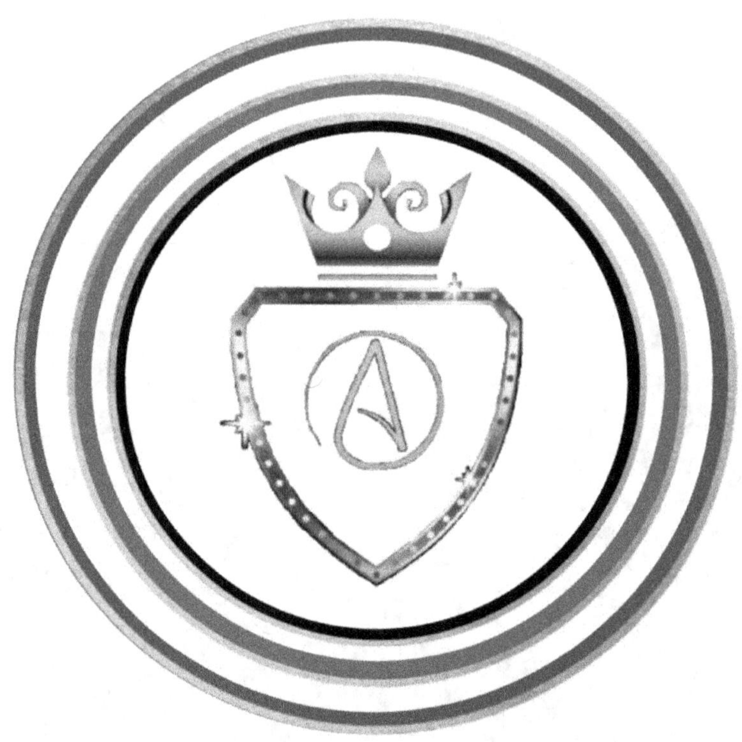

Peace Be With You

Peace Be With You
By: A'nyo Lee

Cover design by: Ataraxis Dynasty Productions
Logo design by: A'nyo Jynnings
Photography by: Ataraxis Dynasty Productions
Edited by:

For Worldwide Distribution
Printed in the United States of America
Published by Ataraxis Dynasty Productions Marketing & Publishing, LLC
Utilizing Microsoft Publishing Software.

Peace Be With You

Peace Be With You

Peace Be With You

Peace Be With You

Peace Be With You

Peace Be With You

To the fathers who stand tall and strong, your presence is a guiding light in our lives. You are the steady anchor, the unwavering support, and the source of boundless love. From teaching us life's valuable lessons to being our rock in times of need, you have shown us the true meaning of strength and dedication. Your sacrifices, both big and small, shape our futures and leave an indelible mark on our hearts. With your gentle words of wisdom and firm yet tender touch, you have nurtured us into the best versions of ourselves. Today and always, we honor and appreciate you, dear fathers, for your unwavering love, unwavering presence, and unwavering commitment to our happiness and well-being.

Dads, countless sacrifices, late-night cooking, projects, cuddles, and heartfelt encouragement sow the seeds of greatness in their children's souls. Their tireless efforts are met with gratitude and admiration from a world that values the transformative power of a loving father. Today, we honor and celebrate these unsung heroes, for their unwavering love and dedication resonate far beyond their own families, shaping a brighter future for all.

A FATHER'S LOVE

A father's love,
Is firm, strong, and true,
Guiding their child to achieve their greatness,
In all they do.
Daddy, with each and every step,
Your wisdom is by my side,
Like the warmth of a constant presence,
Filling up my heartfelt with love, understanding and pride,
Daddy I appreciate you and all you do,
We don't say this enough,
But Daddy we value you for all that you sacrifice,
compromise and do.

.

Peace Be With You

<u>A PROUD CHILD</u>

A tremendous father have patience,
And walk with grace,
A father is firm but yet gentle,
And will always aim to place a smile on your face.
A phenomenal dad may teach you lots of things,
But the beauty of the lesson is always love in self,
A mother's love is priceless,
But a father's love is the root towards logical wealth,
Life can bring the happiest of hearts,
Or unbalanced emotions that would leave you sad,
During these time we don't look for a father,
We yearn for a Dad,
My Hero Through all of life's ups and downs,
You're the Emperor that wears no crown.
Your strength and wisdom light up my way,
Your family is forever grateful,
And this is why everyday with you is Father's Day.

Peace Be With You

A FATHER'S LOVE

Sometimes, people think Fathers are the most ordinary
men,
When they show patience and love,
Father's will fuel your inner purpose,
Just to make sure in Life you rise above,
But what most people don't realize during the turn,
Like heroes, counselors, or story tellers,
They're within your presence to teach but also learn,
The bond shared between a father and child,
It's unbreakable and defining,
Full of Love, logic, and a sense of humor the opposite of
mild,
Dad we appreciate and value you,
Because each day you teach, you protect and you inspire,
You hold with everyone a connection that only grows with
depth,
With a mind that lifts others around you higher,
On this day to be,
Dad we acknowledge all that holds true,
On this very day,
We acknowledge and be grateful for all that you do,
Daddy we love you.

Peace Be With You

SOWING SEEDS

My teacher, my father, my Dad,
I love you for eternity,
My Friend, my logic confidant, and guru,
You're more than just a father to me,
You are beyond just an Emperor,
Dad you are the embodiment of royalty,
The beauty of worldly perfection as much as a man could
be,
No matter how dark things would get,
You make sure you're the one I can always see.
Through laughter and tears,
All of the highs and the lows,
Through the kindness of a father,
Within my mind seeds you sow,
When it comes to loving thy family,
You're the one who truly knows.

Peace Be With You

THE VALUE OF A FATHER'S LOVE

A great dad will always do three things,
And in these three the first is provide,
The second duty of father is to nurture,
While the third is guide,
A father's guidance along your journey,
To make sure you find your way,
To support the family mentally, emotionally, physically,
and financially,
To help all within the fold to seize the day.
Dad, thank you for being there,
And giving Your children more than life,
Your mind ever so strong and wise you see,
But a father's love, no words can suffice.

Peace Be With You

IMAGINATION OF A CHILD

If there is any immortality to be had,
It must be the purity of love from your dad,
No matter what life should ever bring,
A father's job is to uplift your spirits when you're feeling
sad,
A father will let their children fly,
But a dad will let their children soar,
A father would smile at the sight of his kitten,
But a dad will show his child how to roar,
Without question,
Dad you are a hero in my eyes to me,
Dad each day you are a hero,
Brave and strong and who I thrive to be,
Father you are a beacon of light when things go wrong.
Each day, you've shown me the path to be myself and true,
So I am forever grateful,
dear father, I love you.

Peace Be With You

HONOR THY FATHER

Strength and wisdom,
Dad You show empathy within your kindness as you lead
the way,
Without complaining not one time,
You show within your actions daily that everything will be
okay,
Dad, your guiding hand on my shoulder,
Will forever remain,
And the constant lesion you instill within me,
My subconscious will sustain,
Dad, your love is unmatched,
And your strength is a pillar that holds the family up high,
Your spirit replenish our hearts,
And your wisdom is a compass for our minds as the years
fly by,
Thank you, we are forever grateful,
Dad, for all that you do,
On this special day and every day after,
We honor you.

Peace Be With You

SINGING TO MY FATHER

Dad you said,
From the first time the doctor placed me within your arms,
You knew instantly, you'd meet death,
Before you'd let me meet harm,
Dad, I am forever grateful for your love and wisdom,
I'm forever thankful,
For a father like you and the safety of your arms,
I've always felt safe and stable.
You've been my rock through thick and thin,
Your family appreciates you and everything you bring,
On this day we celebrate the strength of you,
Our love for you we sing.

THE GREATEST GIFT

The greatest gift,
The greatest gift I ever had,
Came directly from God,
And I call him dad,
Giving a unconditional love for the family,
Showing the beauty of love with a beautiful variety,
A great father is one of the most unsung, unpraised and
unnoticed,
But yet one of the most valuable assets in our society,
Within the warm clinch of your embrace,
I find solace and peace,
Dad, your love brings comfort towards your children,
And the beauty of a gentle emotional release.
Thank you, Dad,
For simply being there,
Thank you for placing the world upon your shoulders,
And for showing me love and wisdom beyond compare,
Dad, your family appreciates and values you,
As much as the significance of the sun,
Becoming a father is one thing,
But you realized being dad is many things all in one,

Peace Be With You

WE SEE YOUR SACRIFICE

My wise guiding light,
You're the guiding light within your family life's quest,
With the awaiting passion within your love for everyone,
We feel truly honored, at peace, and blessed,
On this day just like the last,
We value you for each sacrifice you make each day,
In order for our family to grow past where it has been,
So, as your family we want to collectively say,
We love and appreciate you more than words can convey.

Peace Be With You

LEGACY

The profound beauty of a father's legacy,
Through your actions through your spark,
Providing the world with gracefulness of a father,
On the beauty of this world you have successfully left a
mark,
Igniting to flames within you,
Driving your admirations forward and never leaving them
idled or in park,
Your strength is unmatched, divine from the start,
As a father you have a legacy that shines even in the dark,
No matter how tough you are, you still showed empathy
and grace,
As a father you've taught your children to be strong, wise
and kind,
A father's love can never be duplicated or replaced,
A father's love to their child 4is forever entwined.

<u>VALUE THY FATHER</u>

A father's unconditional love
Is forever potent within,
A father's heart,
Is patient but firm to build you to win,
A true dad builds love within the heart,
And character within your mind,
A father is always mentally present,
A father's love is kind,
Dad, your love for me knows no bounds,
In your presence we feel uplifted,
And within our heart's happiness surrounds the true
meaning of being profound.
Each day we would like to thank you,
Dad, for all you contentiously do,
We might not acknowledge you or always say it all of the
time,
But dad we value you.

Peace Be With You

<u>WE CELEBRATE YOU</u>

Daddy you are the greatest,
you share your time, effort and energy,
To be a hero to your son's,
And to show your princesses what a true man suppose to
be,
The time spent together,
Manifesting our inner greatness within,
Manifesting the beauty of future memories we've made,
Father and child cruising like batman and robin again,
Drowning in laughter and love that makes life worthwhile.
And very wholesome,
And this is why we celebrate the man you are,
Because of who you are father is why we celebrate ,
Dad, thank you for instilling all of the moments we've
shared,
Forever forming a magnificent bond that's great.

Peace Be With You

MY HEAVENLY GUIDE

I miss you daddy,
With every fiber of my existence to be,
Losing you, caused me to feel as if I lose a piece of myself,
And now all I can do is live within the wisdom you instilled
in me,
Dad, you've been my mentor and guiding star,
Behind you I stride,
Father you calm my soul,
As you encourage me to abandon my pride,
Betting on your family fully in life,
With the sacrifice of each bet,
Dad, you are my emotional doctor and nurturer when my
soul should weep,
Daddy, I aim to walk in your footsteps,
Within your heart I stride,
As we remember every beautiful moment we shared,
And now throughout life you're soul is our guild,
Dad, your courage, wisdom, and knowledge I admire,
So, on this special day like the last,
I want to remind you the love I hold within won't ever
retire.

GRATIFYING LOVE

Dad, you are forever in my heart,
No matter how near or far apart,
You're always with me deep within my spirit,
in how I walk, talk and especially within the beat of my
heart,
A father's love is so divine,
Built with love, courage, wisdom, and empathy,
Just to raise children to be greater than themselves,
So daddy I value the knowledge you had put within me,
The beauty of fathers bond,
The beauty of a bond ever so deep,
A patent love full of warmth and comprehension,
A gratifying love from a father you'll forever keep.

Peace Be With You

<u>A FATHERS DREAM</u>

A father's Dreams,
Forms into the warmth of prosperity,
Deep within the dreams,
Dad, we find inspiration in what could be,
Visions of greatness you instill in each one of us,
The beauty of a future's foundation laid out from your
mind.
Building up the hopes and dreams of your young,
Just so they can expand to be the best versions of
themselves throughout time,
Daddy, you are a guiding swaying light,
Lighting up the darkness within our way,
The beauty of a father's love,
Is now, forever and beyond a day.

Peace Be With You

<u>A FATHERS TEARS</u>

Tears fall for a reason,
And they are your strength not your weakness you see,
The Strength of a Father is internally potent and kind,
A father's strength is divine by time to be,
Unwavering and true the true courage of his mind,
A shield of protection that pulls me through logic and
what's true,
Pouring into value,
As we acknowledge and say thank you,
Greatness without complaining,
Is what a father does for those he adores,
A father's job is to eases the burdens,
of the ones he loves for sure,
Dad, thank you for being my rock,
Whenever I've needed it to be,
I'll cherish the clock,
And time of what you have poured in me.

Peace Be With You

A FATHER'S SMILE

Your smile brightens up my day,
A beacon of joy to the heart,
Lighting up the way.
Thank you, Dad,
For all you say,
Each and every day,
You make sure everyone is okay,
So again we say thank you,
For each and every sacrifice you've made for us,
So dad, to acknowledge your sacrifice,
We celebrate your life with loyalty, love, honesty, and
respect and trust.

Peace Be With You

IN YOUR FOOTSTEPS

I follow in your footsteps,
Strong and sure,
Your guidance and love,
Forever secure.
Thank you,
Dad, for showing me the way,
On this Father's Day,
My love I convey.

A FATHER'S LAUGHTER

Your laughter fills the room with cheer,
A melody that brings joy near.
Thank you,
Dad, for the smiles you bring,
On this special day,
My love I sing.

FEEDING A FATHER SPIRIT

KNOWING YOUR VALUE

No matter what you've been through in your life, Sir, you are worth it. You are worth peace. You are worth to be respected. You are worth, to be able to be vulnerable. And, you are worth to be loved without someone loving the idea of you for what you do for them. You are a phenomenal father, you are a spectacular son, You are valued as a boyfriend, and appreciated as a husband. There's nothing you can't do in life. Conquering everything you want to achieve in your life because you deserve it.

BEING INTENTIONAL

Being intentional with your purpose and moving throughout your purpose intentionality is one of the top ten things that lead to a man's success. Life doesn't give a man its best when a man just waits on it and accept things as they are. We will only go uphill and reach the top pinnacle with intention, discipline, and courage. To improve your life quickly with intention, you must learn to recreate your habits and implant more healthy habits within your day to day routine.

EXCELLENCE OVER PERFECTIONISM

So many of us struggle with perfectionism. It is deep rooted in trepidation and can lead to procrastination. Instead of aiming to be a perfectionist, try focusing more on self excellence, Self-growth, and patience and understanding. Learning within the journey, is part of the process of making something good and then great. You should always aim to leave the best part of yourself in any room or situation you find yourself in. Perfectionism is elusive; it is a state that you can never reach. If you choose excellence over perfectionism, you are choosing progress over constant drive without a direction or purpose. When things are bad we take comfort in the thought they could always be or get worse. And during the rare moments when they are worse, we find hope in the thought that things are so bad they have no other choice to get better. And within those trails, that's when we learn the most from life.

CONTROL YOUR REALITY

It doesn't take a lot to be unforgettable or memorable, but it does take intentionality. What can you say or do to set your experiences apart from others? Think with purpose within each thought, think with positively. Think of all of the possibilities of your future, think of the legacy you are building, and be willing to work for legacy and those possibilities. Aim to be someone who reflects on it happening in your daily realty, this will also help manifest it to happen. Believe it, practice it, and achieve it. Learn to make the possible your reality.

SUCCESS WITHIN YOUR PURPOSE

The greatest leaders are agile and flexible with their patience and understanding. Leaders first chose to lead themselves before they aim to lead others. Men of principal, understands that surprises good and bad, come up in life. People who lead themselves understand the value in having a pre-game plan, but great leaders make halftime adjustments in life they choose to stay flexible and adjust with the day, week, month, or year. By doing this in your life, you will be more successful.

GROW WITH GRACE

There is a gap between where we are, where we want to be, and where we are destined to be. Getting coaching from people who are standing where you are hoping to be helps close this gap. The question you must ask yourself, is what is your growth gap? What will help you close that space and allow your vision to unfold? Get clarity on where you need to grow.

EFFECTIVE CONFIDENT

Effective Father's are confident. They are confident in themselves and believe they can lead people successfully. They are confident in their purpose or mission in life. These father's know what they are doing is needed by the people they want to teach and have lead. They also have confidence in the people they lead and value them greatly.

COMFORT ZONE

Fearlessness is a myth. Instead of trying to be fearless in your day to day life, you should aim to be more brave and understanding. Men who succeed at the highest levels have the same amount of fear as everyone else, but they have learned to be courageous and move forward with courage in the face of fear. Stretch out of your comfort zone little by little each day and aim to be brave!

CHANGE

A man at peace encourages people beneath their umbrella to be positive, motivated people and fans of a peaceful life. A man of peace brings forth extraordinary change within our people lives, which will than bring forth extraordinary change in the man's life. A man at peace will help others to see the possibilities, not problems and the answers, not the questions. What can you look at today that makes you think of positive change. And you sir, are that kind of man.

YOUR COMMUNICATION

Good communicators learn from past circumstances and other great communicators. When observing other great communicators, ask yourself, "How are they connecting healthily with others?" Evaluate how successful communicators connect with people on an empathic and honest level, and then remind yourself, that you can do what they can do. Each day, aim to enhance your understanding and how the way you choose to communicate can affect others. Start watching great communicators, not only listening to what they say to others, but how they say it and connect to them, whether they agree with them or disagree. and you will become a better communicator.

BRANDING

Many believe, if you bring someone in to build your last name and brand, then it will lead to success. But I suggest you first become successful within self first and then brand yourself. Your brand will only be as good as you are, mentally, emotionally, financially, and the self-accountability in your discipline. The best branding is done by the people who have benefited from you being in their life. When they brand you and your name, it is the real thing.

MEDITATION DAILY

Meditate in what brings you peace daily, to preserve what you learned throughout that day. Meditation is our mental processing obstacles in life to keep us from losing ourselves. Finding peace within ourselves, is the first start to leading a peaceful life. When you feel good, you see and experience uplifting things, or instead of feeling good within a moment, you will feel great daily. You immediately file these moments away mentally, so you have access to them when the time is right to uplift yourself again. Meditating, keeps your peace of state and your peace of mind in a calm and relaxed state of being,

BEING RELATABLE

The ability to get along with others and relate to them is a key part in being successful in life. By learning to connect with people and relate with others, your life will be able to reach its full potential pinnacle. The world is full of people thriving to share peace and understanding in their lives. The way you connect to them and how you sustain that very connection will determine how well they'll trust you with their vulnerability, and how much they are willing to help you. Network, connect, and be relatable.

BEING ACCOUNTABLE

It is important for all individuals to have a sense of responsibility, accountability, and take ownership of their own life. You will never do well in life until you take responsibility for your actions or lack of actions and life. You must be accountable for your choices, for who you are within the present moment, for what you do or refuse to do, for your behavior and how you treat others, and how you demand respect from your own self. As a man, responsibility and accountability is a must, because you are expected to be reasonable and accountable for your household,. Take responsibility for the things that happen to you and be accountable for how you treat others in your life.

YOUR ATTITUDE

By parenting with a purpose, you can be the parent that looks at your children and asks how to invest in them correctly without over correcting them and majoring on the minor things in their life. Focusing on attitude, empathy and being a better version of yourself. A good attitude leads to a better life, for you and your children. It is important to have a positive attitude during difficult times and how you handle others. If you are going to succeed in life and want your children to be successful, you need to have the attitude of tenacity to overcome the difficulties in life that everyone experiences with a better perspective and attitude. Attitude is the difference maker. Your attitude will always determine your latitude.

ADDING VALUE

Success is sowing the seeds that benefit others. Success is sowing seeds that don't immediately have a harvest on them. As we are living our lives, we must think and reflect at least once a week, are we sowing seeds for the future and are we adding value to others lives like we would like them to add value to ours? By having an external focus and adding value to yourself and others, the return is far greater than you can ever imagine. But, you will only get this return if you give into your future self and unto others, not just yourself.

INDIVIDUAL SUCCESS

We cannot solve problems with the kind of thinking we engaged when we came up with the problems in the first place. Being a successful starts in your mind first, Being successful is knowing your purpose in life. Until we know why we are here and what we were created for, how can we know we are successful? Money doesn't make you successful, materialistic items doesn't make you successful. Success is finding your purpose in life. The mission is never complete until we find out what is our true calling in life, the calling we have, and the giftedness we have demands that we know what our purpose is. When we know why we are here, that is our purpose, which is the root to our individual success.

A BETTER VERSION

As a man, you should learn as if you will live forever, and live as if you will die tomorrow. The only guarantee in thinking you'll have a better tomorrow, is that you are growing today. You do not go into education, possibilities and opportunities; you grow into education, possibilities and opportunities. This mindset becomes the natural thing to those who keep learning, growing, expanding, and stretching their comfort ones to become a better version of themselves.

ENTHUSIASM

When you give positivity to other people, you get more pleasure in return. You should give a good thought to the happiness and peace you share with others. Pour into people as they are pouring into your life. Live enthusiastically, and be contagious with your enthusiasm. By keeping your dreams alive and creating new dreams and goals, no matter your age and/or stage in life, you can grow the enthusiasm in yourself and others with ease.

PEACE OF STATE

Stay away from those kind of people who try to disparage your ambitions. Small minds will always have small perspectives. But great minds will give you a feeling that you can become even greater too. When you think of leadership within a community, you think of servant leadership. By putting others before yourself and serving those around you, you can become a better leader just by uplifting those in your immediate circle. Growth is essential to lead a peaceful fulfilling life and grow your personal state of being.

MAN OF PURPOSE

When you change your thoughts and perspective in life, remember to also change your habits. Keep in mind; you are the person in charge of your destiny, lead with a true commitment to uplift, educate, and bring prosperity to your life and others through positive uplifting influence. If it is worth doing, it is worth doing right. If you don't do your best, and aim to be your best, one of two things will happen; 1. You'll have to go back and do it over; and 2. If you don't go back and do it, you are shortchanging yourself and those you are trying to lead. As a man of purpose, by doing your best and striving for excellence, you will greatly exceed all of your expectations life.

GODS GIFT

It is only when we take chances within our lives, when our lives improve for the better. The initial and the most difficult risk that we need to take is to become honest with ourselves and keep a healthy balance of self accountability and planning. But the gatekeeper to arrive at self accountability doors is through a higher power than our selves. God is the source and the key. Every good and perfect gift comes from God. The gifts that God has poured into you are greater than you as a whole, and what is more important that the gift itself is what you choose to do with the gift. God, in his purpose for you, gave you those gifts, and it is up to you home in on your gifts, perfect your gifts and pour your gifts back into others. Activate the gifts you are given.

PRIORITIES

Look at your day, and realize that you can't be 100% all the time. You are human, you need breaks. Mental breaks, emotional breaks, physical breaks, But you do need to be 100% on for the things that are priorities in your life. When you look at the teachings of the 4 R's; what is required of you, what gives you the greatest return, what replenish your spirit, and what gives you the greatest reward. If you align those up to find your sweet spot within your priorities, you are on your way. Remember, nature has given you all of the pieces required to achieve exceptional wellness and health, mentally, emotionally, physically, spiritually, and financially, but has left it to you to put these pieces together yourself in discipline.

SELF-AWARENESS

Encouragement is the oxygen of the soul. If you are breathing, you need to be encouraged. A great encourager pours good, motivated, and positive things into other people without expecting anything back in return. A man that pushes encouragement brings to others a sense of peace. No matter, what obstacles they're correctly facing within their own personal lives. A genuine leader is a leader through their actions not just their words, and realizes the current complication is only temporary. A man of true self-awareness realizes that success is not final; failure is not fatal: It is the courage to continue that counts forward.

SELF-CARE

Do you at times beat yourself up? Instead, treat yourself as kindly as you would treat your children, your wife or girlfriend, or even a good friend, if they were dealing with the same challenges you were currently facing or mistake. When we are compassionate towards ourselves and show ourselves empathy, it lowers our stress levels, and help us persevere in life. life is just about living and feeling better about ourselves as we learn and grow within it. Sometimes, it is better to fail in originality than to be successful in imitation and limitations. Your life does not get better by chance, it gets better by change. Change in habits, change in discipline, change in people you surround yourself with, and change in perspective.

KNOW THY SELF

Keep in mind; the road to prosperity and the road to failure are almost exactly the same. A leader is one who, learns the difference between the two paths. A man with a structured mind, learns the way, knows the way, goes the way, and shows the way.

Peace Be With You

RESTORING FAITH IN YOURSELF

Success usually comes to those who are discipline within their actions and who are too busy looking for success and not entertainment. It doesn't pay to get discouraged. Keeping busy and applying confidence in what you are doing, apply grace and understanding to where you are headed, and focus your mindset on a way of life that can once again restore your faith in yourself.

LONGEVITY OR SHORT LIVE

A house won't ever be a home if there is a rivalry between the partners in the home. If you ever find that your house is not a home, you must first start with self and once again become comfortable with yourself and be accountable for where you could do better in the space you are in. Remember, it is easy to place blame on others rather than changing thy self, but what comes easy is always the most difficult during the longevity of it all.

YOUR MINDSET IS KEY

Developing a successful mindset from the swift teachings of your failures. Discouragement and failure are two of the surest stepping stones towards success. Stop waiting for everything to be perfect before you decide to enjoy your life. Learn to celebrate the small victories in your life as much as you want to celebrate the major victories.

EDUCATE YOURSELF

Nothing in the world can take the place of discipline and persistence. Talent will not; nothing is more common than unsuccessful men with talent. Genius will not; unrewarded genius is almost a proverb. Education will not; the world is full of educated derelicts. The slogan 'Keep moving forward' has solved and always will solve the problems of where a man needs growth in his life. Never let the fear of striking out get in your way. Always conquer your legacy daily, you are and will always be worth it.

EMPATHY

Optimism is a happiness and success magnet. If you stay positive, good things and good people will be drawn to you. There are three ways to ultimate success: The first way is to be kind. The second way is to show empathy. The third way is to handle others with grace and mercy.

SELF SENTIMENT

Success within self is peace of mind, which is a direct result of self-satisfaction in knowing you made the effort to become the best of which you are capable, within that day, week, month, or year. Success within self is a constant and consistent sentiment. A person with a clear purpose and seek out the meaning behind their purpose, will make progress on even the roughest road. A person with no purpose will make no progress on even the smoothest of days.

DREAM OR WORK

You should never dream about success. You should always aim to work for it and earn it in your daily discipline and actions. What's for you is for you but the only way to obtain your success is by putting forth the effort and keep moving forward, even if it looks like you are going nowhere. You got this; you need to believe it to achieve it.

BELIEVE IT AND YOU'LL ACHIEVE IT

A naysayer sees the difficulty in every opportunity; an optimist sees the opportunity in every difficulty. Each day the choice is yours, to be a Optimistic person or live in negativity as a pessimistic individual.
Keep in mind; success is getting what you want; but happiness is wanting what you get.

<u>UPLIFT ME NOT</u>

Don't be afraid of change because it is leading you to new beginnings. Life shrinks or expands in proportion to one's perspective, habits, discipline, and courage. Never let yesterday take up too much of today.

IT TAKES WORK

Growth does not simply happen to us by chance. We have to choose growth and keep choosing it every day. Whether that grow is self-growth, financial growth, mental and/or emotional growth and so on. You learn more from failure than from success. Don't let failure, shortcomings, or setbacks stop you from moving forward towards your success. Failure builds character.

ALTERING REALITY

If you are working on something that you really care about,
you don't have to be motivated or pushed. The vision pulls
you towards the journey of it daily. There are three ways of
meeting difficulties: You alter the difficulties, you alter
yourself to meet what's needed to conquer the difficulties,
or you let the difficulties discourage you.

MOVING FORWARD

Between you and every goal that you wish to achieve, there
is a series of obstacles, and the bigger the goal, the bigger
the obstacles. Moving toward the obstacles and keeping the
focus of what you are thriving to achieve brings experience.
And experience is a hard teacher because she gives the test
first, the lesson afterwards.

FEEDING YOUR AMBITION

The only limit to our realization of tomorrow will be our doubts of today. To know how much there is to know is the beginning of learning to live life and live in it rather than just being alive with no purpose of your own to accomplish. Setting goals is the secret to a compelling future. Little goals turn into bigger goals and bigger goals turns into colossal goals. Each ambition should be a step towards an even greater aspiration in the future.

<u>LEARN TO CONCENTRATE</u>

When we long for life without difficulties, remind us that
oaks grow strong in contrary winds and diamonds are made
under pressure. Learn to concentrate all your thoughts upon
the work in hand. The sun's rays do not burn until brought
to a focus. At times, we must accept restricted displeasure,
but we should never lose infinite hope within our dream
and purpose.

Peace Be With You

Peace Be With You

Present fathers, whether they live with their children or not, are the most unsung heroes of our lives. Dads, play an irreplaceable role in shaping the future of their children. They are the guiding lights and the pillars of strength within the household. And the unwavering support that every child needs growing up in a curious world full of misinformation. A phenomenal father is more than just a biological presence; he is a mentor, a role model, and a source of unconditional love for his children. His influence extends far beyond the walls of the house, because a father's influence will always turn a house into a home. A father's gentle but firm love impact more than just his family, reaching out and touching the lives of not only his children but also the world around them.

In a society that sometimes underestimates the significance of fatherhood, it is imperative to acknowledge and appreciate these remarkable individuals who embrace their responsibilities with passion, empathy, patience, and dedication. The world recognizes the immense impact that fathers have on the development and well-being of their children and family, and it celebrates their unwavering commitment. Their dedication inspires and empowers the next generation and every generation afterwards, fostering a sense of security, resilience, and compassion. Let us cherish and honor these phenomenal fathers like yourself, for they and you are the foundations upon which greatness is built.

Peace Be With You

Peace Be With You

Thank you for reading

Peace Be With You

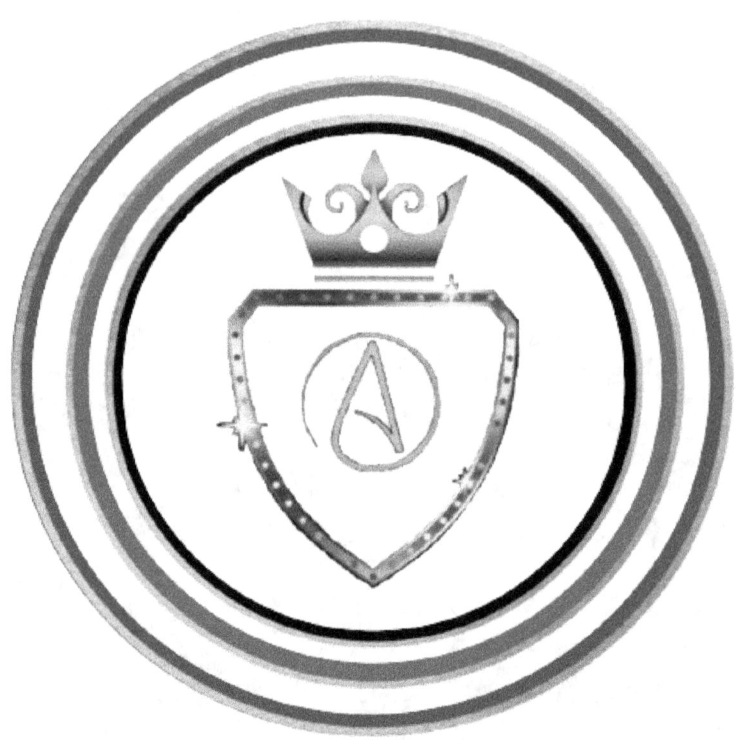

Peace Be With You

Peace Be With You

More Books from A'nyo Lee:

The Drug Game Street politics
A Strange Mind
Secrets of Eden
Secrets of Eden 2
Secrets of Eden 3
Panty Dropper
Mirror Image
Life of emotions
Life of emotions 2
Beyond the Smoke
I am training to be great
Mommy there is a zoo in my room
The Exchange
A Dynamic Of Change
See through Dragon Eyes
The Fairy and the Frog
The rose inside of my Heart
Redrum Deadly Devotion
Redrum heavy Rain
Redrum The Art of Devotion
Redrum Odyssey of the Mind
I Don't Know Who Needs Free Game
Monogamy Isn't For Me

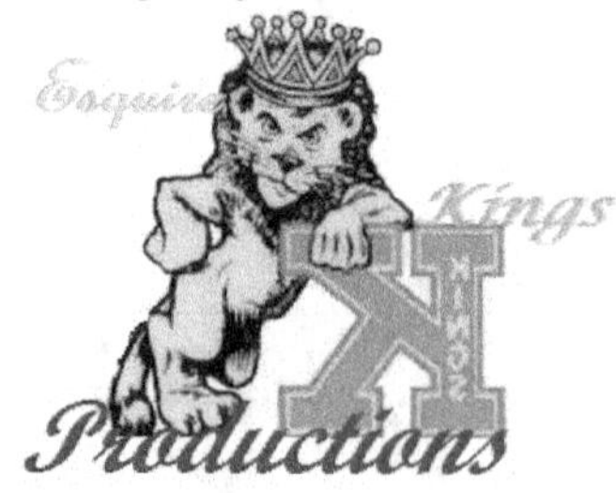

More Books from A'nyo Lee:

The Unapologetic Gentlemen-An Ace Dangerous Thirst
The Unapologetic Gentlemen-The Devil's Gift
The Unapologetic Gentlemen-Sin And Sinuous
The Unapologetic Gentlemen-Empire Of Spades
Narcissistic Behavior
The Shadowkeeper
My Beautiful Ether Within
Perspective
So You Think You're Poly
Poetry In Motion
The Book Of Patience
The Night Of the Living
Ataraxis Dynasty-Manifesting Society Secrets
The Roots Of A Revolution
A Moment In Time
Beautiful Lies
Sexual Seduction
Beautiful Reflection
The Children of the Emperor
Peace Be With You
Enthrall Solitude

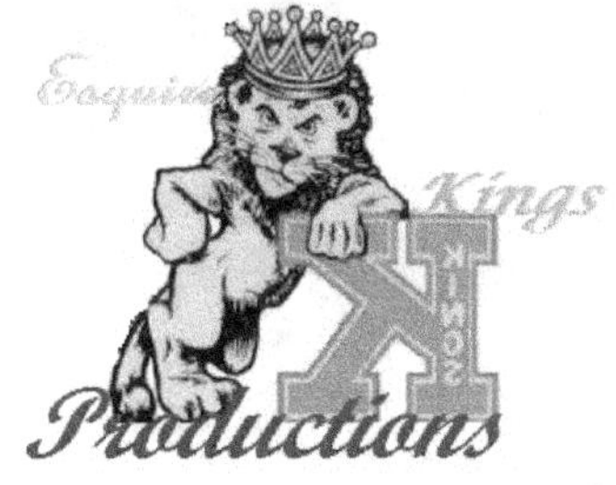

Peace Be With You